DATE

SYMPTOMS

cramping	muscle pain	seizures
anxiety	nerve pain	headache
fatigue	joint pain	dizziness
depression	nausea	eye pressure
appetite loss	stress	spasms
	other _____	

product used _____

dosage _____

method _____

other meds _____

NOTES

Did your symptoms improve, stay the same, or get worse?

DATE

SYMPTOMS

cramping	muscle pain	seizures
anxiety	nerve pain	headache
fatigue	joint pain	dizziness
depression	nausea	eye pressure
appetite loss	stress	spasms

other _____

product used _____

dosage _____

method _____

other meds _____

NOTES

Did your symptoms improve, stay the same, or get worse?

DATE

SYMPTOMS

cramping	muscle pain	seizures
anxiety	nerve pain	headache
fatigue	joint pain	dizziness
depression	nausea	eye pressure
appetite loss	stress	spasms

other _____

product used _____

dosage _____

method _____

other meds _____

NOTES

Did your symptoms improve, stay the same, or get worse?

DATE

SYMPTOMS

cramping	muscle pain	seizures
anxiety	nerve pain	headache
fatigue	joint pain	dizziness
depression	nausea	eye pressure
appetite loss	stress	spasms

other _____

product used _____

dosage _____

method _____

other meds _____

NOTES

Did your symptoms improve, stay the same, or get worse?

DATE

SYMPTOMS

cramping	muscle pain	seizures
anxiety	nerve pain	headache
fatigue	joint pain	dizziness
depression	nausea	eye pressure
appetite loss	stress	spasms

other _____

product used _____

dosage _____

method _____

other meds _____

NOTES

Did your symptoms improve, stay the same, or get worse?

DATE

SYMPTOMS

cramping	muscle pain	seizures
anxiety	nerve pain	headache
fatigue	joint pain	dizziness
depression	nausea	eye pressure
appetite loss	stress	spasms

other _____

product used _____

dosage _____

method _____

other meds _____

NOTES

Did your symptoms improve, stay the same, or get worse?

DATE

SYMPTOMS

cramping	muscle pain	seizures
anxiety	nerve pain	headache
fatigue	joint pain	dizziness
depression	nausea	eye pressure
appetite loss	stress	spasms

other _____

product used _____

dosage _____

method _____

other meds _____

NOTES

Did your symptoms improve, stay the same, or get worse?

DATE

SYMPTOMS

cramping	muscle pain	seizures
anxiety	nerve pain	headache
fatigue	joint pain	dizziness
depression	nausea	eye pressure
appetite loss	stress	spasms

other _____

product used _____

dosage _____

method _____

other meds _____

NOTES

Did your symptoms improve, stay the same, or get worse?

DATE

SYMPTOMS

cramping	muscle pain	seizures
anxiety	nerve pain	headache
fatigue	joint pain	dizziness
depression	nausea	eye pressure
appetite loss	stress	spasms

other _____

product used _____

dosage _____

method _____

other meds _____

NOTES

Did your symptoms improve, stay the same, or get worse?

DATE

SYMPTOMS

cramping	muscle pain	seizures
anxiety	nerve pain	headache
fatigue	joint pain	dizziness
depression	nausea	eye pressure
appetite loss	stress	spasms

other _____

product used _____

dosage _____

method _____

other meds _____

NOTES

Did your symptoms improve, stay the same, or get worse?

DATE

SYMPTOMS

cramping	muscle pain	seizures
anxiety	nerve pain	headache
fatigue	joint pain	dizziness
depression	nausea	eye pressure
appetite loss	stress	spasms

other _____

product used _____

dosage _____

method _____

other meds _____

NOTES

Did your symptoms improve, stay the same, or get worse?

DATE

SYMPTOMS

cramping	muscle pain	seizures
anxiety	nerve pain	headache
fatigue	joint pain	dizziness
depression	nausea	eye pressure
appetite loss	stress	spasms

other _____

product used _____

dosage _____

method _____

other meds _____

NOTES

Did your symptoms improve, stay the same, or get worse?

DATE

SYMPTOMS

cramping	muscle pain	seizures
anxiety	nerve pain	headache
fatigue	joint pain	dizziness
depression	nausea	eye pressure
appetite loss	stress	spasms

other _____

product used _____

dosage _____

method _____

other meds _____

NOTES

Did your symptoms improve, stay the same, or get worse?

DATE

SYMPTOMS

cramping	muscle pain	seizures
anxiety	nerve pain	headache
fatigue	joint pain	dizziness
depression	nausea	eye pressure
appetite loss	stress	spasms

other _____

product used _____

dosage _____

method _____

other meds _____

NOTES

Did your symptoms improve, stay the same, or get worse?

DATE

SYMPTOMS

cramping	muscle pain	seizures
anxiety	nerve pain	headache
fatigue	joint pain	dizziness
depression	nausea	eye pressure
appetite loss	stress	spasms

other _____

product used _____

dosage _____

method _____

other meds _____

NOTES

Did your symptoms improve, stay the same, or get worse?

DATE

SYMPTOMS

cramping	muscle pain	seizures
anxiety	nerve pain	headache
fatigue	joint pain	dizziness
depression	nausea	eye pressure
appetite loss	stress	spasms

other _____

product used _____

dosage _____

method _____

other meds _____

NOTES

Did your symptoms improve, stay the same, or get worse?

DATE

SYMPTOMS

cramping	muscle pain	seizures
anxiety	nerve pain	headache
fatigue	joint pain	dizziness
depression	nausea	eye pressure
appetite loss	stress	spasms

other _____

product used _____

dosage _____

method _____

other meds _____

NOTES

Did your symptoms improve, stay the same, or get worse?

DATE

SYMPTOMS

cramping	muscle pain	seizures
anxiety	nerve pain	headache
fatigue	joint pain	dizziness
depression	nausea	eye pressure
appetite loss	stress	spasms

other _____

product used _____

dosage _____

method _____

other meds _____

NOTES

Did your symptoms improve, stay the same, or get worse?

DATE

SYMPTOMS

cramping	muscle pain	seizures
anxiety	nerve pain	headache
fatigue	joint pain	dizziness
depression	nausea	eye pressure
appetite loss	stress	spasms

other _____

product used _____

dosage _____

method _____

other meds _____

NOTES

Did your symptoms improve, stay the same, or get worse?

DATE

SYMPTOMS

cramping	muscle pain	seizures
anxiety	nerve pain	headache
fatigue	joint pain	dizziness
depression	nausea	eye pressure
appetite loss	stress	spasms

other _____

product used _____

dosage _____

method _____

other meds _____

NOTES

Did your symptoms improve, stay the same, or get worse?

DATE

SYMPTOMS

cramping	muscle pain	seizures
anxiety	nerve pain	headache
fatigue	joint pain	dizziness
depression	nausea	eye pressure
appetite loss	stress	spasms

other _____

product used _____

dosage _____

method _____

other meds _____

NOTES

Did your symptoms improve, stay the same, or get worse?

DATE

SYMPTOMS

cramping	muscle pain	seizures
anxiety	nerve pain	headache
fatigue	joint pain	dizziness
depression	nausea	eye pressure
appetite loss	stress	spasms

other _____

product used _____

dosage _____

method _____

other meds _____

NOTES

Did your symptoms improve, stay the same, or get worse?

DATE

SYMPTOMS

cramping	muscle pain	seizures
anxiety	nerve pain	headache
fatigue	joint pain	dizziness
depression	nausea	eye pressure
appetite loss	stress	spasms

other _____

product used _____

dosage _____

method _____

other meds _____

NOTES

Did your symptoms improve, stay the same, or get worse?

DATE

SYMPTOMS

cramping	muscle pain	seizures
anxiety	nerve pain	headache
fatigue	joint pain	dizziness
depression	nausea	eye pressure
appetite loss	stress	spasms

other _____

product used _____

dosage _____

method _____

other meds _____

NOTES

Did your symptoms improve, stay the same, or get worse?

DATE

SYMPTOMS

cramping	muscle pain	seizures
anxiety	nerve pain	headache
fatigue	joint pain	dizziness
depression	nausea	eye pressure
appetite loss	stress	spasms

other _____

product used _____

dosage _____

method _____

other meds _____

NOTES

Did your symptoms improve, stay the same, or get worse?

DATE

SYMPTOMS

cramping	muscle pain	seizures
anxiety	nerve pain	headache
fatigue	joint pain	dizziness
depression	nausea	eye pressure
appetite loss	stress	spasms

other _____

product used _____

dosage _____

method _____

other meds _____

NOTES

Did your symptoms improve, stay the same, or get worse?

DATE

SYMPTOMS

cramping	muscle pain	seizures
anxiety	nerve pain	headache
fatigue	joint pain	dizziness
depression	nausea	eye pressure
appetite loss	stress	spasms

other _____

product used _____

dosage _____

method _____

other meds _____

_____

NOTES

_____

Did your symptoms improve, stay the same, or get worse?

DATE

SYMPTOMS

cramping	muscle pain	seizures
anxiety	nerve pain	headache
fatigue	joint pain	dizziness
depression	nausea	eye pressure
appetite loss	stress	spasms

other _____

product used _____

dosage _____

method _____

other meds _____

NOTES

Did your symptoms improve, stay the same, or get worse?

DATE

SYMPTOMS

cramping	muscle pain	seizures
anxiety	nerve pain	headache
fatigue	joint pain	dizziness
depression	nausea	eye pressure
appetite loss	stress	spasms

other _____

product used _____

dosage _____

method _____

other meds _____

NOTES

Did your symptoms improve, stay the same, or get worse?

DATE

SYMPTOMS

cramping	muscle pain	seizures
anxiety	nerve pain	headache
fatigue	joint pain	dizziness
depression	nausea	eye pressure
appetite loss	stress	spasms

other _____

product used _____

dosage _____

method _____

other meds _____

NOTES

Did your symptoms improve, stay the same, or get worse?

DATE

SYMPTOMS

cramping	muscle pain	seizures
anxiety	nerve pain	headache
fatigue	joint pain	dizziness
depression	nausea	eye pressure
appetite loss	stress	spasms
	other _____	

product used _____

dosage _____

method _____

other meds _____

NOTES

Did your symptoms improve, stay the same, or get worse?

DATE

SYMPTOMS

cramping	muscle pain	seizures
anxiety	nerve pain	headache
fatigue	joint pain	dizziness
depression	nausea	eye pressure
appetite loss	stress	spasms

other _____

product used _____

dosage _____

method _____

other meds _____

NOTES

Did your symptoms improve, stay the same, or get worse?

DATE

SYMPTOMS

cramping	muscle pain	seizures
anxiety	nerve pain	headache
fatigue	joint pain	dizziness
depression	nausea	eye pressure
appetite loss	stress	spasms

other _____

product used _____

dosage _____

method _____

other meds _____

NOTES

Did your symptoms improve, stay the same, or get worse?

DATE

SYMPTOMS

cramping	muscle pain	seizures
anxiety	nerve pain	headache
fatigue	joint pain	dizziness
depression	nausea	eye pressure
appetite loss	stress	spasms

other _____

product used _____

dosage _____

method _____

other meds _____

NOTES

Did your symptoms improve, stay the same, or get worse?

DATE

SYMPTOMS

cramping	muscle pain	seizures
anxiety	nerve pain	headache
fatigue	joint pain	dizziness
depression	nausea	eye pressure
appetite loss	stress	spasms

other _____

product used _____

dosage _____

method _____

other meds _____

NOTES

Did your symptoms improve, stay the same, or get worse?

DATE

SYMPTOMS

cramping	muscle pain	seizures
anxiety	nerve pain	headache
fatigue	joint pain	dizziness
depression	nausea	eye pressure
appetite loss	stress	spasms

other _____

product used _____

dosage _____

method _____

other meds _____

NOTES

Did your symptoms improve, stay the same, or get worse?

DATE

SYMPTOMS

cramping	muscle pain	seizures
anxiety	nerve pain	headache
fatigue	joint pain	dizziness
depression	nausea	eye pressure
appetite loss	stress	spasms
	other _____	

product used _____

dosage _____

method _____

other meds _____

NOTES

Did your symptoms improve, stay the same, or get worse?

DATE

SYMPTOMS

cramping	muscle pain	seizures
anxiety	nerve pain	headache
fatigue	joint pain	dizziness
depression	nausea	eye pressure
appetite loss	stress	spasms

other _____

product used _____

dosage _____

method _____

other meds _____

NOTES

Did your symptoms improve, stay the same, or get worse?

DATE

SYMPTOMS

cramping	muscle pain	seizures
anxiety	nerve pain	headache
fatigue	joint pain	dizziness
depression	nausea	eye pressure
appetite loss	stress	spasms

other _____

product used _____

dosage _____

method _____

other meds _____

NOTES

Did your symptoms improve, stay the same, or get worse?

DATE

SYMPTOMS

cramping	muscle pain	seizures
anxiety	nerve pain	headache
fatigue	joint pain	dizziness
depression	nausea	eye pressure
appetite loss	stress	spasms

other _____

product used _____

dosage _____

method _____

other meds _____

NOTES

Did your symptoms improve, stay the same, or get worse?

DATE

SYMPTOMS

cramping	muscle pain	seizures
anxiety	nerve pain	headache
fatigue	joint pain	dizziness
depression	nausea	eye pressure
appetite loss	stress	spasms
	other _____	

product used _____

dosage _____

method _____

other meds _____

NOTES

Did your symptoms improve, stay the same, or get worse?

DATE

SYMPTOMS

cramping	muscle pain	seizures
anxiety	nerve pain	headache
fatigue	joint pain	dizziness
depression	nausea	eye pressure
appetite loss	stress	spasms

other _____

product used _____

dosage _____

method _____

other meds _____

NOTES

Did your symptoms improve, stay the same, or get worse?

DATE

SYMPTOMS

cramping	muscle pain	seizures
anxiety	nerve pain	headache
fatigue	joint pain	dizziness
depression	nausea	eye pressure
appetite loss	stress	spasms
	other _____	

product used _____

dosage _____

method _____

other meds _____

NOTES

Did your symptoms improve, stay the same, or get worse?

DATE

SYMPTOMS

cramping	muscle pain	seizures
anxiety	nerve pain	headache
fatigue	joint pain	dizziness
depression	nausea	eye pressure
appetite loss	stress	spasms

other _____

product used _____

dosage _____

method _____

other meds _____

NOTES

Did your symptoms improve, stay the same, or get worse?

DATE

SYMPTOMS

cramping	muscle pain	seizures
anxiety	nerve pain	headache
fatigue	joint pain	dizziness
depression	nausea	eye pressure
appetite loss	stress	spasms

other _____

product used _____

dosage _____

method _____

other meds _____

NOTES

Did your symptoms improve, stay the same, or get worse?

DATE

SYMPTOMS

cramping	muscle pain	seizures
anxiety	nerve pain	headache
fatigue	joint pain	dizziness
depression	nausea	eye pressure
appetite loss	stress	spasms

other _____

product used _____

dosage _____

method _____

other meds _____

NOTES

Did your symptoms improve, stay the same, or get worse?

DATE

SYMPTOMS

cramping	muscle pain	seizures
anxiety	nerve pain	headache
fatigue	joint pain	dizziness
depression	nausea	eye pressure
appetite loss	stress	spasms

other _____

product used _____

dosage _____

method _____

other meds _____

NOTES

Did your symptoms improve, stay the same, or get worse?

DATE

SYMPTOMS

cramping	muscle pain	seizures
anxiety	nerve pain	headache
fatigue	joint pain	dizziness
depression	nausea	eye pressure
appetite loss	stress	spasms

other _____

product used _____

dosage _____

method _____

other meds _____

NOTES

Did your symptoms improve, stay the same, or get worse?

DATE

SYMPTOMS

cramping	muscle pain	seizures
anxiety	nerve pain	headache
fatigue	joint pain	dizziness
depression	nausea	eye pressure
appetite loss	stress	spasms

other _____

product used _____

dosage _____

method _____

other meds _____

NOTES

Did your symptoms improve, stay the same, or get worse?

DATE

SYMPTOMS

cramping	muscle pain	seizures
anxiety	nerve pain	headache
fatigue	joint pain	dizziness
depression	nausea	eye pressure
appetite loss	stress	spasms

other _____

product used _____

dosage _____

method _____

other meds _____

NOTES

Did your symptoms improve, stay the same, or get worse?

DATE

SYMPTOMS

cramping	muscle pain	seizures
anxiety	nerve pain	headache
fatigue	joint pain	dizziness
depression	nausea	eye pressure
appetite loss	stress	spasms

other _____

product used _____

dosage _____

method _____

other meds _____

NOTES

Did your symptoms improve, stay the same, or get worse?

DATE

SYMPTOMS

cramping	muscle pain	seizures
anxiety	nerve pain	headache
fatigue	joint pain	dizziness
depression	nausea	eye pressure
appetite loss	stress	spasms

other _____

product used _____

dosage _____

method _____

other meds _____

NOTES

Did your symptoms improve, stay the same, or get worse?

DATE

SYMPTOMS

cramping	muscle pain	seizures
anxiety	nerve pain	headache
fatigue	joint pain	dizziness
depression	nausea	eye pressure
appetite loss	stress	spasms

other _____

product used _____

dosage _____

method _____

other meds _____

NOTES

Did your symptoms improve, stay the same, or get worse?

DATE

SYMPTOMS

cramping	muscle pain	seizures
anxiety	nerve pain	headache
fatigue	joint pain	dizziness
depression	nausea	eye pressure
appetite loss	stress	spasms

other _____

product used _____

dosage _____

method _____

other meds _____

NOTES

Did your symptoms improve, stay the same, or get worse?

DATE

SYMPTOMS

cramping	muscle pain	seizures
anxiety	nerve pain	headache
fatigue	joint pain	dizziness
depression	nausea	eye pressure
appetite loss	stress	spasms
	other _____	

product used _____

dosage _____

method _____

other meds _____

NOTES

Did your symptoms improve, stay the same, or get worse?

DATE

SYMPTOMS

cramping	muscle pain	seizures
anxiety	nerve pain	headache
fatigue	joint pain	dizziness
depression	nausea	eye pressure
appetite loss	stress	spasms

other _____

product used _____

dosage _____

method _____

other meds _____

NOTES

Did your symptoms improve, stay the same, or get worse?

DATE

SYMPTOMS

cramping	muscle pain	seizures
anxiety	nerve pain	headache
fatigue	joint pain	dizziness
depression	nausea	eye pressure
appetite loss	stress	spasms

other _____

product used _____

dosage _____

method _____

other meds _____

NOTES

Did your symptoms improve, stay the same, or get worse?

DATE

SYMPTOMS

cramping	muscle pain	seizures
anxiety	nerve pain	headache
fatigue	joint pain	dizziness
depression	nausea	eye pressure
appetite loss	stress	spasms

other _____

product used _____

dosage _____

method _____

other meds _____

NOTES

Did your symptoms improve, stay the same, or get worse?

DATE

SYMPTOMS

cramping	muscle pain	seizures
anxiety	nerve pain	headache
fatigue	joint pain	dizziness
depression	nausea	eye pressure
appetite loss	stress	spasms

other _____

product used _____

dosage _____

method _____

other meds _____

NOTES

Did your symptoms improve, stay the same, or get worse?

DATE

SYMPTOMS

cramping	muscle pain	seizures
anxiety	nerve pain	headache
fatigue	joint pain	dizziness
depression	nausea	eye pressure
appetite loss	stress	spasms

other _____

product used _____

dosage _____

method _____

other meds _____

NOTES

Did your symptoms improve, stay the same, or get worse?

DATE

SYMPTOMS

cramping	muscle pain	seizures
anxiety	nerve pain	headache
fatigue	joint pain	dizziness
depression	nausea	eye pressure
appetite loss	stress	spasms

other _____

product used _____

dosage _____

method _____

other meds _____

NOTES

Did your symptoms improve, stay the same, or get worse?

DATE

SYMPTOMS

cramping	muscle pain	seizures
anxiety	nerve pain	headache
fatigue	joint pain	dizziness
depression	nausea	eye pressure
appetite loss	stress	spasms

other _____

product used _____

dosage _____

method _____

other meds _____

NOTES

Did your symptoms improve, stay the same, or get worse?

DATE

SYMPTOMS

cramping	muscle pain	seizures
anxiety	nerve pain	headache
fatigue	joint pain	dizziness
depression	nausea	eye pressure
appetite loss	stress	spasms

other _____

product used _____

dosage _____

method _____

other meds _____

NOTES

Did your symptoms improve, stay the same, or get worse?

DATE

SYMPTOMS

cramping	muscle pain	seizures
anxiety	nerve pain	headache
fatigue	joint pain	dizziness
depression	nausea	eye pressure
appetite loss	stress	spasms

other _____

product used _____

dosage _____

method _____

other meds _____

NOTES

Did your symptoms improve, stay the same, or get worse?

DATE

SYMPTOMS

cramping	muscle pain	seizures
anxiety	nerve pain	headache
fatigue	joint pain	dizziness
depression	nausea	eye pressure
appetite loss	stress	spasms

other _____

product used _____

dosage _____

method _____

other meds _____

NOTES

Did your symptoms improve, stay the same, or get worse?

DATE

SYMPTOMS

cramping	muscle pain	seizures
anxiety	nerve pain	headache
fatigue	joint pain	dizziness
depression	nausea	eye pressure
appetite loss	stress	spasms

other _____

product used _____

dosage _____

method _____

other meds _____

NOTES

Did your symptoms improve, stay the same, or get worse?

DATE

SYMPTOMS

cramping	muscle pain	seizures
anxiety	nerve pain	headache
fatigue	joint pain	dizziness
depression	nausea	eye pressure
appetite loss	stress	spasms
	other _____	

product used _____

dosage _____

method _____

other meds _____

NOTES

Did your symptoms improve, stay the same, or get worse?

DATE

SYMPTOMS

cramping	muscle pain	seizures
anxiety	nerve pain	headache
fatigue	joint pain	dizziness
depression	nausea	eye pressure
appetite loss	stress	spasms

other _____

product used _____

dosage _____

method _____

other meds _____

NOTES

Did your symptoms improve, stay the same, or get worse?

DATE

SYMPTOMS

cramping	muscle pain	seizures
anxiety	nerve pain	headache
fatigue	joint pain	dizziness
depression	nausea	eye pressure
appetite loss	stress	spasms

other _____

product used _____

dosage _____

method _____

other meds _____

NOTES

Did your symptoms improve, stay the same, or get worse?

DATE

SYMPTOMS

cramping	muscle pain	seizures
anxiety	nerve pain	headache
fatigue	joint pain	dizziness
depression	nausea	eye pressure
appetite loss	stress	spasms

other _____

product used _____

dosage _____

method _____

other meds _____

NOTES

Did your symptoms improve, stay the same, or get worse?

DATE

SYMPTOMS

cramping	muscle pain	seizures
anxiety	nerve pain	headache
fatigue	joint pain	dizziness
depression	nausea	eye pressure
appetite loss	stress	spasms

other _____

product used _____

dosage _____

method _____

other meds _____

NOTES

Did your symptoms improve, stay the same, or get worse?

DATE

SYMPTOMS

cramping	muscle pain	seizures
anxiety	nerve pain	headache
fatigue	joint pain	dizziness
depression	nausea	eye pressure
appetite loss	stress	spasms

other _____

product used _____

dosage _____

method _____

other meds _____

NOTES

Did your symptoms improve, stay the same, or get worse?

DATE

SYMPTOMS

cramping	muscle pain	seizures
anxiety	nerve pain	headache
fatigue	joint pain	dizziness
depression	nausea	eye pressure
appetite loss	stress	spasms

other _____

product used _____

dosage _____

method _____

other meds _____

NOTES

Did your symptoms improve, stay the same, or get worse?

DATE

SYMPTOMS

cramping	muscle pain	seizures
anxiety	nerve pain	headache
fatigue	joint pain	dizziness
depression	nausea	eye pressure
appetite loss	stress	spasms

other _____

product used _____

dosage _____

method _____

other meds _____

NOTES

Did your symptoms improve, stay the same, or get worse?

DATE

SYMPTOMS

cramping	muscle pain	seizures
anxiety	nerve pain	headache
fatigue	joint pain	dizziness
depression	nausea	eye pressure
appetite loss	stress	spasms

other _____

product used _____

dosage _____

method _____

other meds _____

NOTES

Did your symptoms improve, stay the same, or get worse?

DATE

SYMPTOMS

cramping	muscle pain	seizures
anxiety	nerve pain	headache
fatigue	joint pain	dizziness
depression	nausea	eye pressure
appetite loss	stress	spasms

other _____

product used _____

dosage _____

method _____

other meds _____

NOTES

Did your symptoms improve, stay the same, or get worse?

DATE

SYMPTOMS

cramping	muscle pain	seizures
anxiety	nerve pain	headache
fatigue	joint pain	dizziness
depression	nausea	eye pressure
appetite loss	stress	spasms
	other _____	

product used _____

dosage _____

method _____

other meds _____

NOTES

Did your symptoms improve, stay the same, or get worse?

DATE

SYMPTOMS

cramping	muscle pain	seizures
anxiety	nerve pain	headache
fatigue	joint pain	dizziness
depression	nausea	eye pressure
appetite loss	stress	spasms

other _____

product used _____

dosage _____

method _____

other meds _____

NOTES

Did your symptoms improve, stay the same, or get worse?

DATE

SYMPTOMS

cramping	muscle pain	seizures
anxiety	nerve pain	headache
fatigue	joint pain	dizziness
depression	nausea	eye pressure
appetite loss	stress	spasms

other _____

product used _____

dosage _____

method _____

other meds _____

NOTES

Did your symptoms improve, stay the same, or get worse?

DATE

SYMPTOMS

cramping	muscle pain	seizures
anxiety	nerve pain	headache
fatigue	joint pain	dizziness
depression	nausea	eye pressure
appetite loss	stress	spasms

other _____

product used _____

dosage _____

method _____

other meds _____

NOTES

Did your symptoms improve, stay the same, or get worse?